MENOPAUSE:

FREQUENT QUESTIONS AND ANSWERS

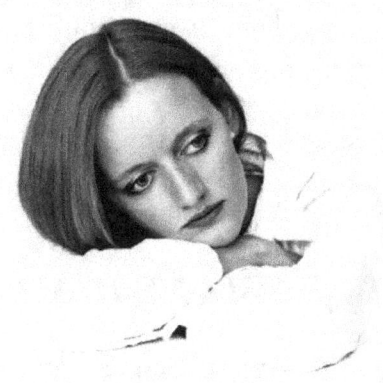

Berna Vermont
Elsa Markeys
Susy Mora
Monica Parker
Daniel Parson

Vermont Indie Books

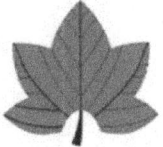

GRAPEVINE BOOKS
2015

DISCLAIMER

Published by: Ediciones De La Parra

A WORD FROM THE AUTHOR

This book presents the most frequent questions and answers regarding menopause, its causes, symptoms and treatments.

I´d like to thank the team of writers that made this book possible: Elsa Markeys, Susy Mora, Mónica Parker and Daniel Parson, whose generous research and writings fill these pages and without whom this book would never have seen public light.

Berna Vermont

ISBN-13: 978-1522789963

ISBN-10:1522789960

TABLE OF CONTENTS:

WHAT IS MENOPAUSE?

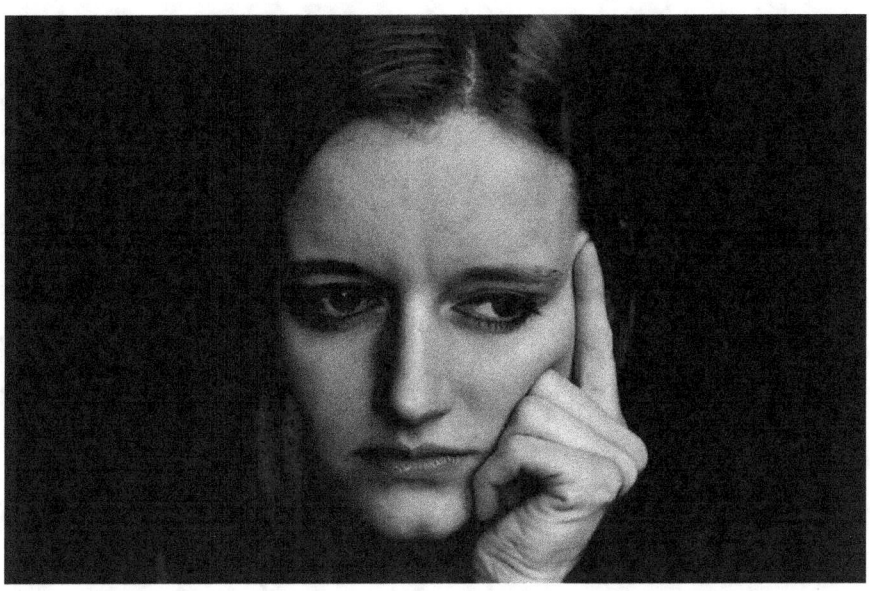

According to the National Institute on Aging (NIA), nearly 2 million U.S. women will turn 50 this year. And most of these females are experiencing or will experience the symptoms of perimenopause, menopause or post-menopause, three stages in a woman´s life that are bound to affect their physical and mental functions if not properly treated.

Menopause can be defined as a three-stage phase in every woman´s life that marks the end of her fertile, reproductive years. It usually manifests fully when females turns 50, affecting them differently according to their genetic inheritance and their past and present lifestyles, including their daily diet, physical activity, addictions, and mental health.

Scientifically, menopause is caused by a progressive drop in the levels of female hormones like estrogen and progesterone (also known as progestin), which gradually begin to decrease once they reach middle age, affecting them physically and mentally.

It must be said that estrogen and progesterone are vital for women in their fertile years. A drop in their levels produces irregular periods with shorter, longer, heavier or lighter cycles, ultimately leading to the cessation of menstruation and producing dramatic long-term physical and mental consequences if not treated properly.

WHAT ARE THE THREE STAGES OF MENOPAUSE?

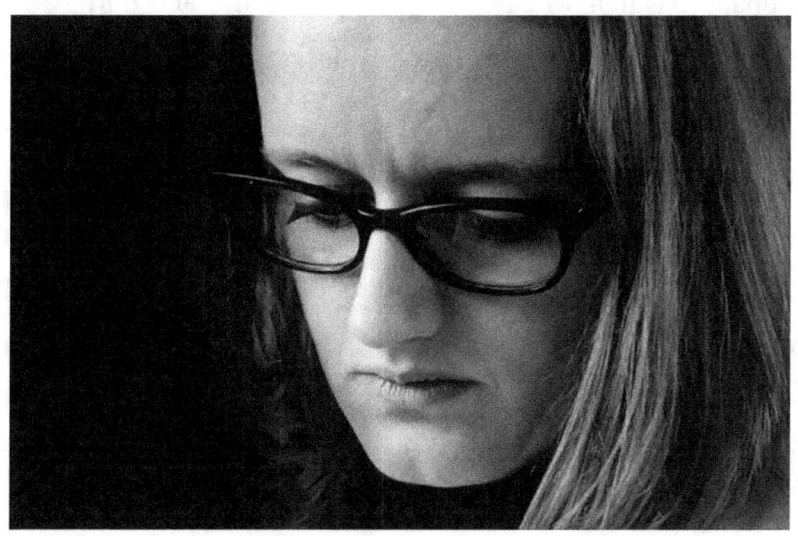

The three stages of menopause are the following:

1:PERIMENOPAUSE:

This first stage, also known as "the prelude to menopause", generally starts when a woman is in her mid-forties, producing irregularities in the frequency, intensity and duration of her menstrual cycles and causing a series of unwanted physical and emotional symptoms that can last from 5 to 10 years.

Perimenopause begins with a drop in female hormone levels, changing the frequency, duration and intensity of a woman´s menstrual cycle which in spite of having been always regular, suddenly becomes unpredictable. Once she goes 12 months without menstruating, it is said that she has officially reached menopause. And, after this, she enters the stage of post-menopause, which will last the rest of her life and during which she may become prone to certain diseases, including bone loss (osteoporosis) and heart disease.

2:MENOPAUSE:

After going through the long years of perimenopause, in which a woman´s menstrual cycle become more and more infrequent, it is said that a woman officially reaches menopause once she has gone a full 12 months without menstruating (usually around 50 years of age).

3:POST-MENOPAUSE:

Once menopause has been reached a woman becomes permanently infertile and thus begins a new stage known as post-menopause, which will last for the rest of her life. Without proper treatment, during this last phase she may become prone to certain physical disorders, mainly bone loss (osteoporosis) and heart disease.

Although many women experience severe symptoms during their perimenopause, menopause and post-menopause, a small percentage of women pass these stages without experiencing any symptoms.

HOW MANY WOMEN ARE MENOPAUSIC?

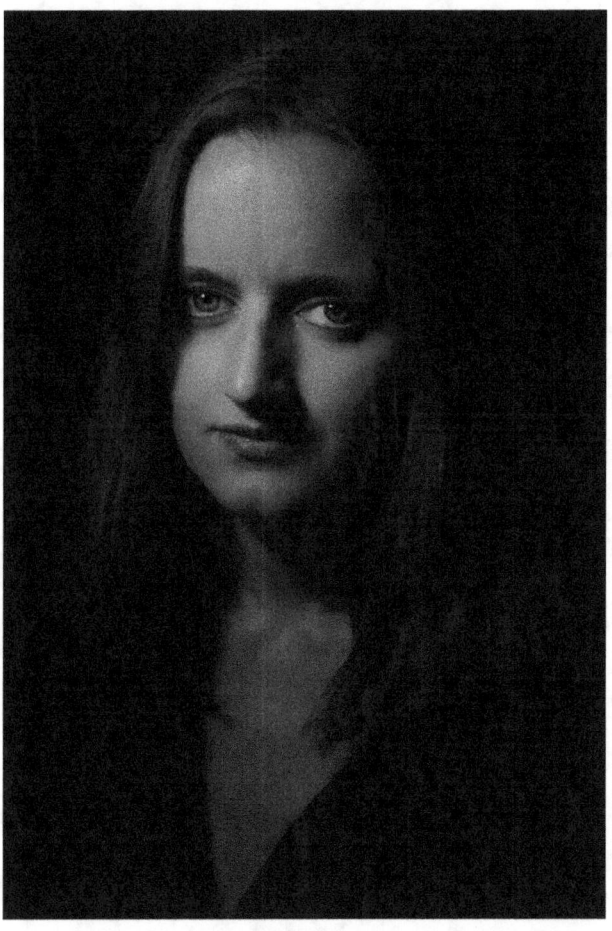

According to the National Institute on Aging (NIA), nearly 2 million U.S. women will turn 50 this year. And most of these females are presently experiencing or are bound to experience the symptoms of perimenopause, menopause and post-menopause, three stages in a woman´s life that can affect their physical and mental functions if not properly treated.

The following are some of the latest facts and figures released by the North American Menopause Society (NAMS):

-Each day approximately 6,000 US females reach the age of menopause (on average around age 51). This equals over 2 million women each year.

-Over 6 out of 10 US females experiencing peri-menopause and menopause symptoms understand these as "natural transitions".

-Thanks to menopause remedies, 8 out of 10 US females experiencing menopause report no significant decrease in their quality of life.

-About half of US females experiencing menopause report no significant loss of sex drive.

-Approximately 5 out of 10 women experiencing post-menopause report being happier than in their 40s, 30s and 20s.

IS IT PRE-MENOPAUSE OR PERIMENOPAUSE?

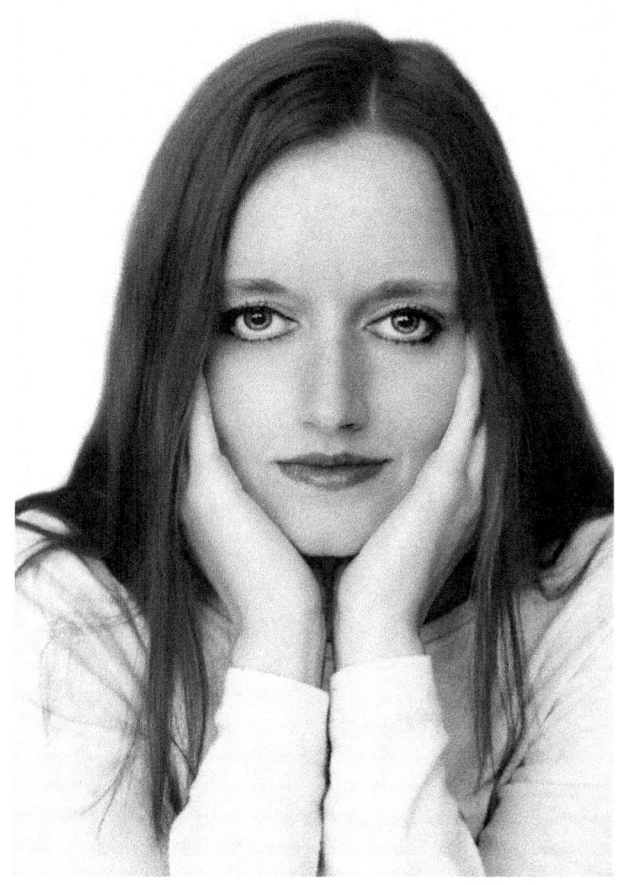

Some people mistakenly use the term *pre-menopause* ("before menopause") when referring to the stage immediately before menopause. Why is this a mistake?

First of all, according to medical science *pre-menopause* refers to the initial stage in a woman′s reproductive life, from the day she has her first period (during puberty) to the time she has her first menopause symptoms, including hot flashes, night sweats and mood swings, among others.

Secondly, because the stage that begins when a female first experiences these symptoms, that is, the stage immediately before menopause, is actually called *perimenopause* ("around menopause"). It usually begins when she is in her 40s and ends once she definitely stops menstruating, marking the end of her reproductive life.

WHICH ARE THE MOST-COMMON MENOPAUSE MYTHS?

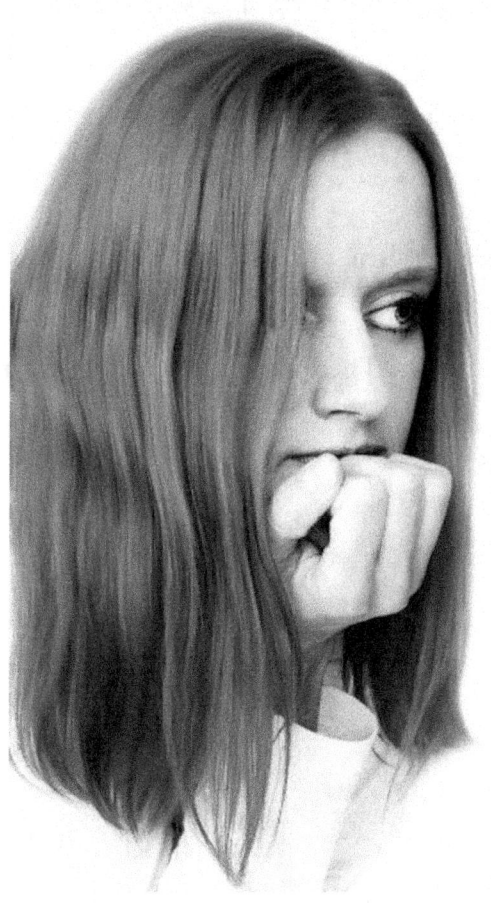

The following are the three most-common menopause myths or mistaken beliefs:

1: **Menopause is an illness**: Menopause is a natural phase of life that affects ALL women in their 40s and 50s, not an illness or disease.

2: **Menopause is the end of a woman´s productive life:** By no means this is true. Actually, a large percentage of the 50 million North American women currently facing menopause are active, productive workers.

3: **Menopause means "the end is near":** According to the U. S. Census, average life expectancy is presently at 78, with many living in their 80s and 90s. There, when women reach menopause they often have several decades of life ahead.

WHICH ARE THE 35 SYMPTOMS OF MENOPAUSE?

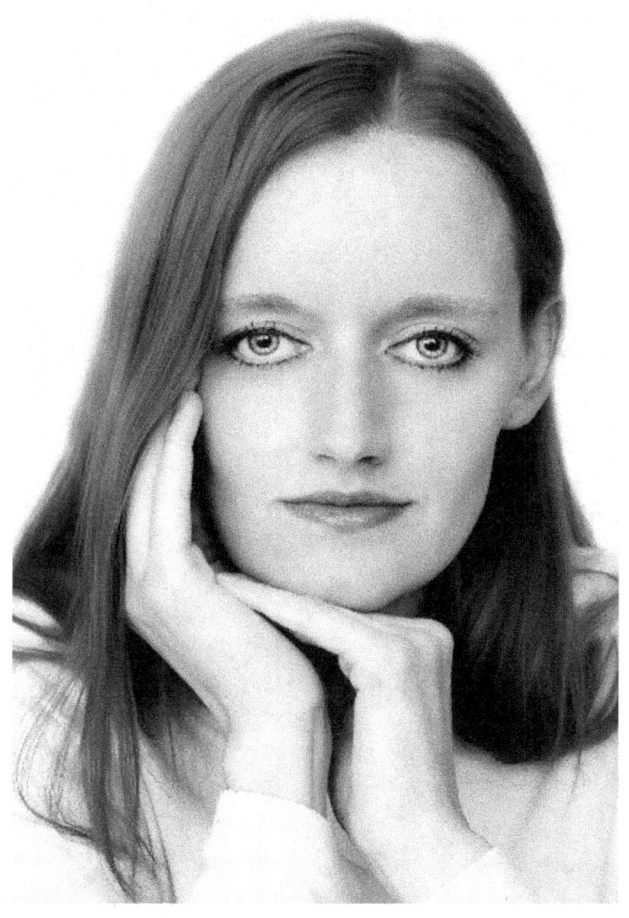

The following are the 35 most-common peri-menopause, menopause and post-menopause symptoms identified by medical science:

1-Hot flashes

2-Night sweats

3-Mood swings

4-Irritability

5-Depression

6-Loss of sex drive

7- Loss of memory and concentration (Brain Fog)

8-Allergy symptoms

9-Breast tenderness

10-Chronic fatigue

11-Unstable blood sugar levels

12-Dizziness, lightheadedness

13-Dry, thin or wrinkly skin

14-Endometriosis

15-Facial hair growth

16-Fibrocystic breasts

17-Thinning hair, hair loss, brittle nails

18 -Headaches (migraines)

19-Heart palpitations.

20-Heavy or light menstruation

21-Incontinence

22 -Irregular periods

23-Leg cramps

24-Tingling or cold extremities

25-Low metabolism

26-Menstrual cramps

27-Osteoporosis

28-Tinnitus: Ringing or buzzing in ears

29-Insomnia (sleep disorder)

30-Spotting, light bleeding

31-Hypothyroidism symptoms

32-Urinary tract and yeast infections

33-Uterine fibroids

34 - Water retention and weight gain

35-Lightheadedness or dizziness

WHICH ARE THE MOST FREQUENT SYMPTOMS?

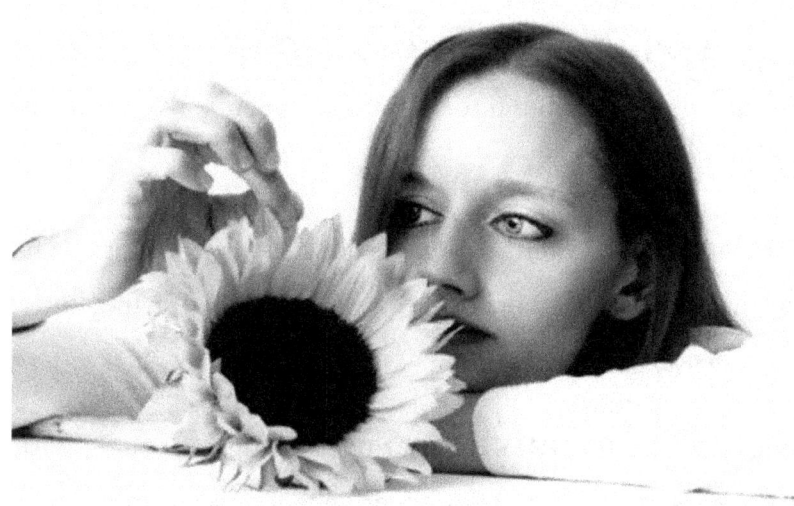

Alth ough a small percentage of women are fortunate enough to go through the three stages of menopause without showing any critical symptoms, most of them experience minor or major troubles with at least one or more of the following:

HOT FLASHES: Scientifically known as vasomotor symptoms (VMS), they are experienced as a wave of intense heat that lasts from a couple of minutes to half an hour or more, producing sweating and faster heartbeat rates.

NIGHT SWEATS: Hot flashes during sleep produce what is known as "night sweats", usually interrupting sleep and causing insomnia and tiredness.

IRRITABILITY: Hormonal fluctuations may also cause bad temper, popularly known as crankiness or "bitchy attitude" for no apparent reason.

BRAIN FOG: Described as memory loss and lack of concentration, this symptom threatens the productive lives of a vast percentage of women.

DEPPRESSION: Some women experience intense and recurring sadness for no apparent reason, mostly affecting those with a past history of depression.

LOSS OF SEX DRIVE: During menopause and post-menopause most women –not all- experience vaginal dryness and a lack of sexual desire.

ANXIETY: Drops in hormone levels and the inability to cope with aging and change produce in some women "anxiety attacks" for no apparent reason.

HEADACHES: Hormone drops can cause headaches or menstrual migraines in women who reach perimenopause -even if they've never had them.

More details about these symptoms and how to fight them in the following chapters.

WHAT IS HORMONE REPLACEMENT THERAPY?

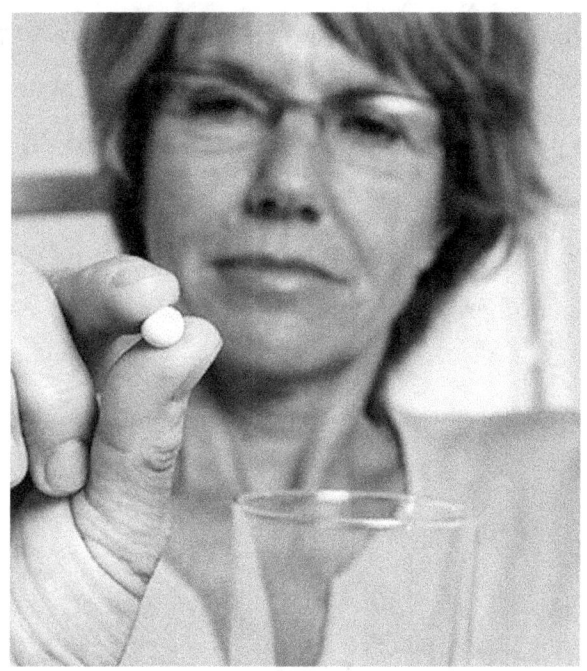

Back in the 1940s, scientists found that female hormones can be taken artificially to ease perimenopausal, menopausal and post-menopausal symptoms. This medical practice is known as Hormone Replacement Therapy or HRT.

Up to the early twenty-first century, most doctors prescribed hormone replacement therapy (HRT) to ease menopause symptoms. However, in 2002, the United States National Institutes of Health (NIH) showed that prolonged HRT actually boosts the risk of heart disease, stroke, breast cancer, and blood clots, causing more disease than it prevents. Jesus! Just think of the thousands of women who took this therapy over the last decades and died due to this unprecedented "scientific mistake"!

Presently, an increasing number of doctors are prescribing dietary supplements and herbal products together with a balanced diet, proper exercise and lifestyle changes to fight menopause symptoms. They focus on 100% natural treatments that have proven to be effective and without side effects, including dietary supplements and herbal extracts.

IS MENOPAUSE A GOOD OR BAD PHASE IN LIFE?

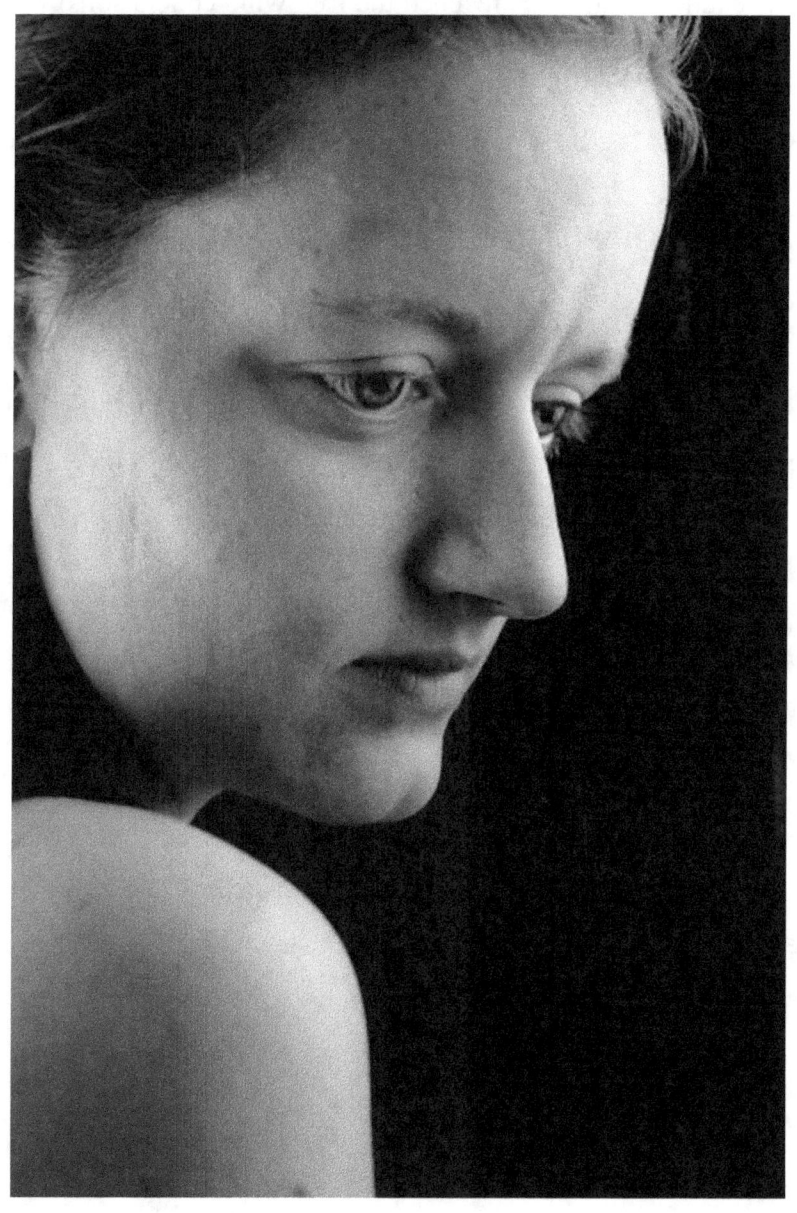

According to the Department of Clinical Neuroscience of the Karolinska Institute (Stockholm, Sweden), after studying the psychological development of 130 healthy, menopausal women for 5 consecutive years, they reached the following conclusions:

-Initially, most participants (57%) had neutral beliefs about menopause.

-Initially, at least 31% were pessimistic about menopause.

-Initially, only 12% were optimistic about menopause.

A closer look revealed that the optimistic and neutral females experienced "lighter" menopause symptoms, whereas the pessimistic experienced "heavier" ones.

Surprisingly, over the 5-year period most neutral and pessimistic women turned optimistic:

-In their last interviews, up to 67% appraised menopause positively.

In conclusion, most females ended up being optimistic about menopause! Everything indicates that these women over the years discovered, like Cybill Shepherd said, that menopause *"is not easy, but it is also another exciting stage!"*

DO I NEED PROFESSIONAL TREATMENT?

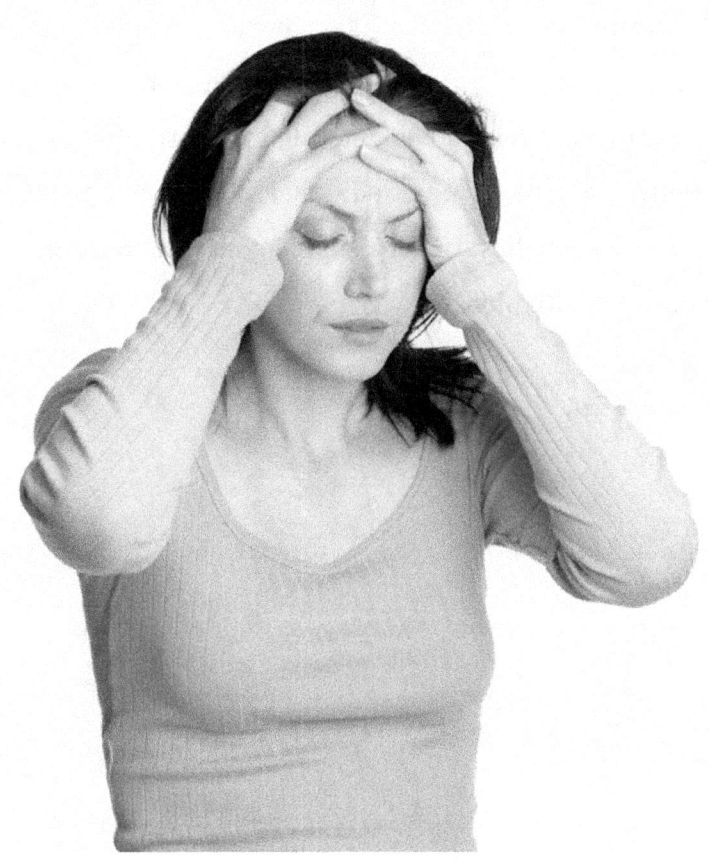

According to the Mayo Clinic, with proper medical treatment and supervision, women *"can stay healthy, vital and sexual"* during the years of menopause, which they define as *"the natural biological process marking the permanent end of menstruation and fertility"*.

Mayo Clinic specialists recommend preventive health care during and after menopause, as well as a series of physical screenings including thyroid testing, colonoscopy, lipid screening, and mammography, as well as breast and pelvic exams.

A word of advice: If you're presently experiencing perimenopause, menopause or post-menopause symptoms, see your doctor and take advantage of the many effective treatments presently available, from traditional hormone therapy to natural menopause remedies, dietary supplements, exercise programs and preventive health plans!

WHAT ARE HOT FLASHES?

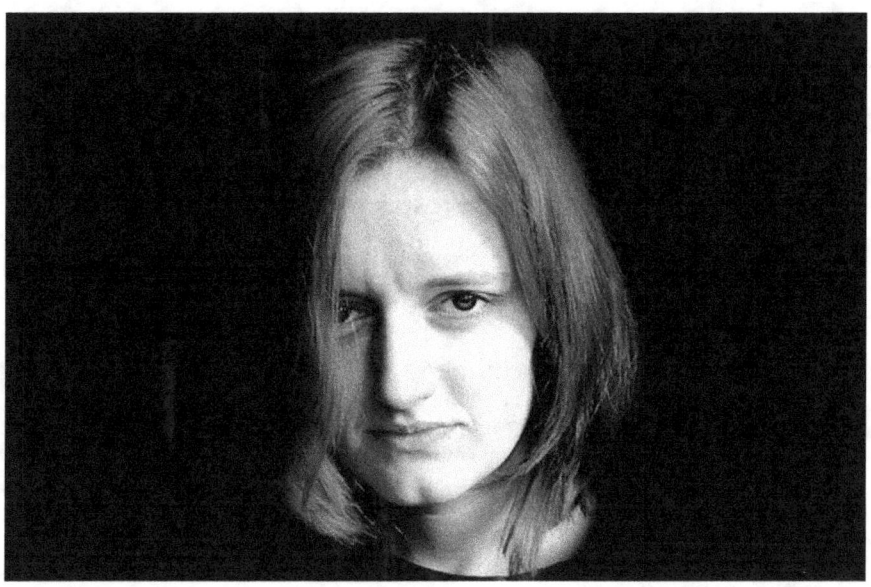

A hot flash is like a wave of sudden fever spreading through the body, usually affecting the head and neck regions and causing immediate perspiration and flushing.

Although it is believed that hot flashes are the effect of decreasing estrogen levels, to this date scientists still haven´t found its true physical causes.

Most women facing perimenopause and menopause experience recurring hot flashes (up to 80% in their fifth year and down to 10% ten years after reaching menopause)

They often come at night, interrupting sleep and causing night sweats, insomnia and daytime tiredness.

They come in different intensities and generally last from brief seconds to a few minutes.

They affect women as well as their bed partners, generating sleep deprivation and causing daytime tiredness in both partners.

According to a Cochrane Prospective Meta-Analysis (PMA), oral hormone therapy (estrogens only or estrogens with progesterone) is highly effective in diminishing hot flashes. Nevertheless, with the declining use of hormone replacement therapy, natural products have recently become the best alternative for women seeking to decrease the recurrence and intensity of hot flashes in a safe and healthy way.

WHAT IS PREMATURE MENOPAUSE?

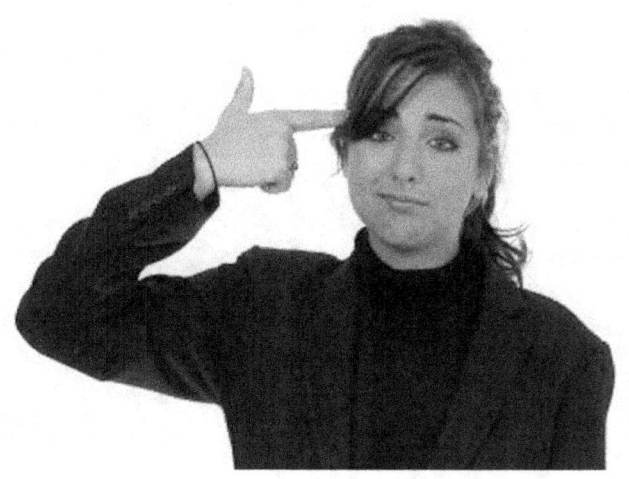

If you are under 40 and are experiencing menopause symptoms like hot flashes and mood swings, you may be experiencing premature or early menopause. Although this condition affects a relatively small percentage of females under the age of 40, it´s relatively common in young women that have undergone chemotherapy or radiation treatment, have a genetic predisposition or suffer autoimmune disorders like hypothyroidism, Grave´s disease or lupus.

As in the case of other females experiencing menopause, this condition is characterized by lower estrogen levels, affecting overall health and increasing the chances of osteoporosis, heart problems and gum disease, among other health issues. Therefore, if you are under 40 and are experiencing menopause symptoms, my best advice is to see your doctor for professional advice.

WHAT ABOUT PREVENTING PREAGNANCY?

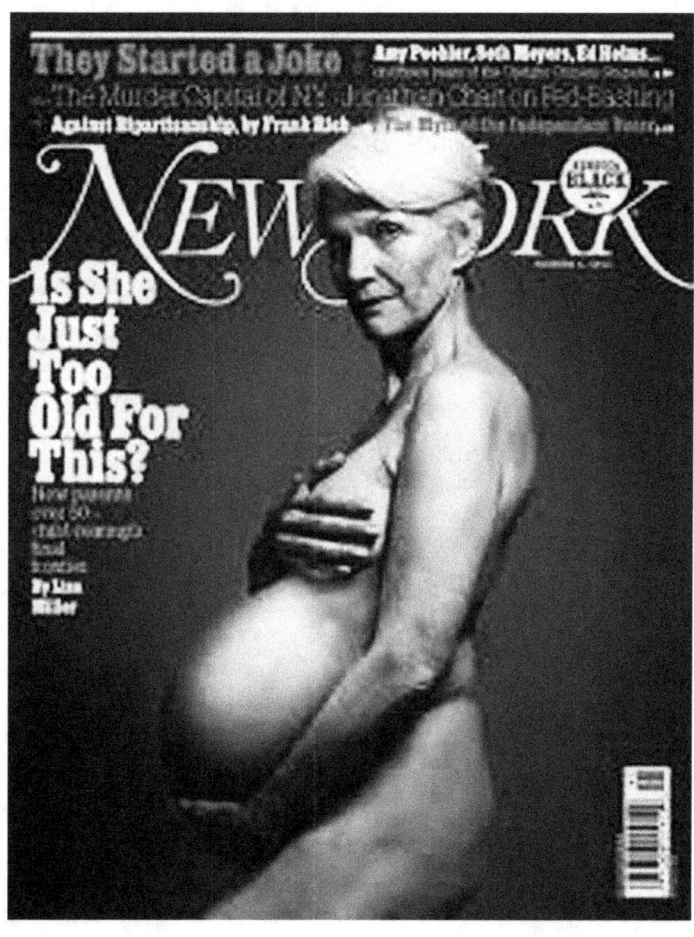

¿Can you get pregnant during menopause? ¿What are the odds?

According to doctor Margery Gass, Executive Director of the North American Menopause Society (NAMS), getting pregnant during menopause is absolutely possible, although the odds are relatively small: less than one percent.

"Pregnancy is always a possibility unless you´ve gone a whole year without a period," he explained, "so never assume that you can´t get pregnant even if you´re experiencing menopausal symptoms like hot flashes or have skipped periods for several months."

For birth control during menopause, doctor Gass recommends an intrauterine device (IUD) or low-dose birth control pills, which not only prevent pregnancy but can also ease menopause symptoms like hot flashes and mood swings.

IS MENOPAUSE AFFECTING YOUR WORK?

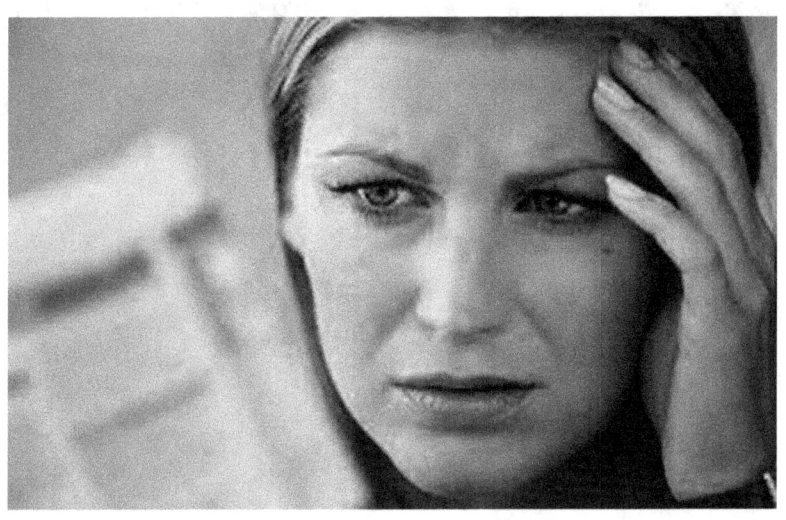

If the menopause is affecting your work, you are not alone. There are approximately three and a half million women over 50 currently holding a job in the United States. Almost half of these women (45%) find their symptoms hard to deal with, harming their working performance and relationships with co-workers. At least 35% experience bearable symptoms , mostly hot flashes, night sweats, irritability, mood swings, brain fog, and depression. The remaining 20% have almost no symptoms (apart from less-frequent periods that eventually stop altogether),

Unfortunately, most employers are not aware that women in their perimenopause, menopause and post-menopause often need special consideration. In result, most females hide their condition, coping with their symptoms in silence. In fact, according to a study conducted by the University of Nottingham, most women are *"little prepared for the arrival of the menopause, and even less equipped to manage its symptoms at work... Over half had not disclosed their symptoms to their manager."*

HOW TO AVOID WEIGHT GAIN DURING MENOPAUSE?

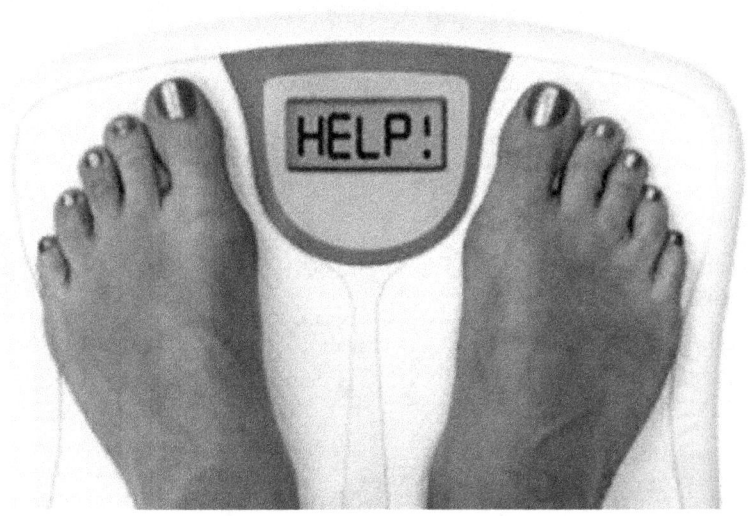

One of the unwanted symptoms us women face during menopause is a decrease in muscle mass. This means fewer calories are needed to keep our bodies functioning and therefore less food is required to meet our regular energy levels. So, if you don´t change your eating habits, you will surely experience weight gain (like I did).

To avoid weight gain during "the years of change", apart from taking natural menopause remedies and changing your eating habits, I recommend thirty minutes of fast walking per day, which made me lose 15lb (7kg) over the last 12 months and also helped me reduce the frequency and intensity of hot flashes and night sweats, among other menopause symptoms. Be well!

WHAT IS THE IMPORTANCE OF A HEALTHY DIET?

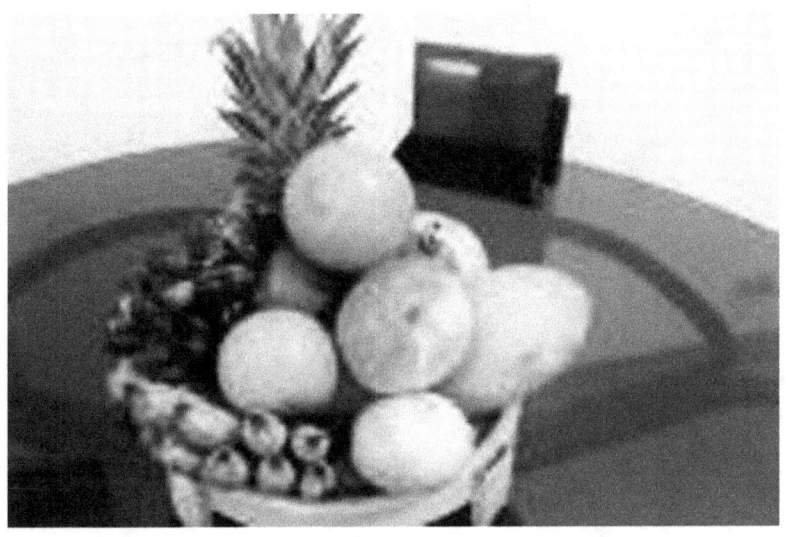

Together with menopause supplements and a "hale and hearty" lifestyle, a healthy diet can help you reduce menopause symptoms. But, what is a healthy diet and how can it help me?

A healthy diet is often defined as a "good, balanced diet". It´s basically "all you can eat to improve your health and general wellbeing".

In the case of women going through menopause, like you and me, a healthy diet must include dietary and menopause supplements to help us prevent weight gain and reduce symptoms like hot flashes, night sweats, mood swings, , poor concentration, irritability, headaches and heavy or irregular menstruations.

So, if you´re going through menopause follow my advice: Make the necessary diet and lifestyle changes as soon as you can and improve your health and natural well-being! After all, if I did it then why can´t you?

HOW CAN I ASSURE A HEALTHY DIET?

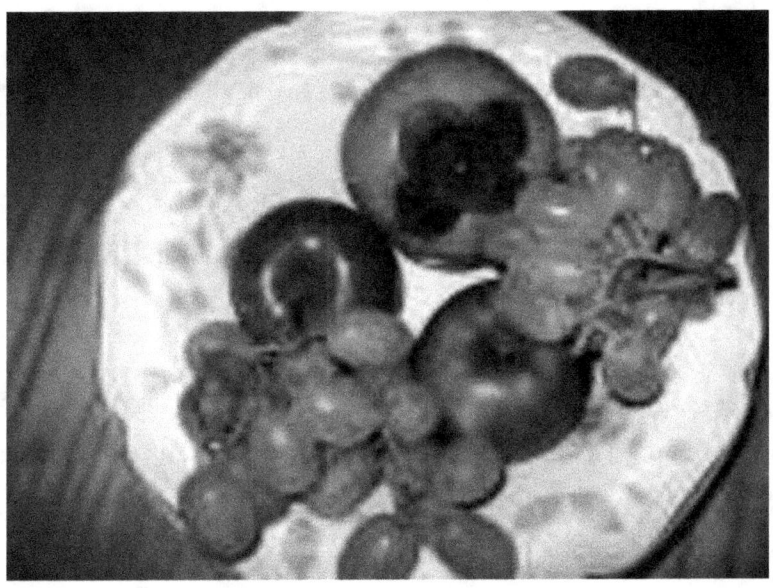

The following tips are most useful when planning a healthy diet:

Always grill instead of frying your food.

Make sure to drink only semi-skimmed, 1% or skimmed milk.

Always opt for low or reduced-fat dairy products.

Cut down on salt and avoid processed foods.

Always eat plenty of fruits and vegetables, as well as oats, wholegrain cereals and beans.

Vitamin D is very important and is found in cereals, eggs, red meat, oily fish, cod liver oil, and fortified margarine, among other foods.

Regarding the loss of calcium that affects women as they approach menopause, causing osteoporosis, scientists have found that many natural nutrients can help to maintain healthy calcium levels, including fruit and vegetables as well as foods from the milk and dairy group, for these provide calcium. Also a must are calcium supplements.

Due to the fact that during menopause and post-menopause the risk of heart disease may increase, your diet should include less saturated and trans fats and more lean cuts of meat, without excess fat, avoiding processed meat products.

Keep away from sodas and junk food (including fast-food). A healthy diet will help you prevent the weight gain triggered during the perimenopause and menopause, when most women lose muscle mass and therefore their bodies need less calories to survive.

See a specialist. Remember that this book is for educational purposes only and is not recommended as a means of diagnosing or treating your specific condition. If you are experiencing perimenopause, menopause, or post-menopause symptoms and need treatment and a healthy diet planned especially for your particular case, please consult your physician or nutritionist.

WHAT ARE MENOPAUSE SUPPLEMENTS?

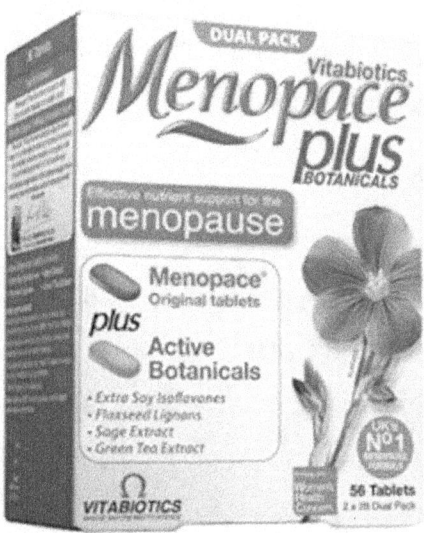

An increasing number of women are turning to natural menopause therapies based on dietary supplements and herbal products to help females through "the long and winding" years of menopause.

Menopause supplements, such as **Femestron** for example, are also known as "**natural menopause remedies**" and are sold over-the-counter (without prescription) in the form of pills that only need to be taken once or twice a day.

The most effective contain chromium, niacin, black cohosh, red clover, chasteberry, and soybean isoflavones, among other 100%

natural ingredients proven to relieve the most common peri-menopause, menopause and post-menopause symptoms, mainly hot flashes, night sweats, mood swings, depression, irritability, diminished energy, and loss of sex drive.

Together with a balanced diet, regular exercise plus a healthy lifestyle, menopause supplements, as in my case, will literally change your life!

One of the most effective ingredients contained in the leading menopause supplements, including Femestron, is wild yam *(Dioscorea villosa)*. This plant has been used for centuries by herbalists to treat menstrual cramps and digestive problems, and is presently believed to increase progesterone levels in females.

WHAT ARE NATURAL MENOPAUSE REMEDIES?

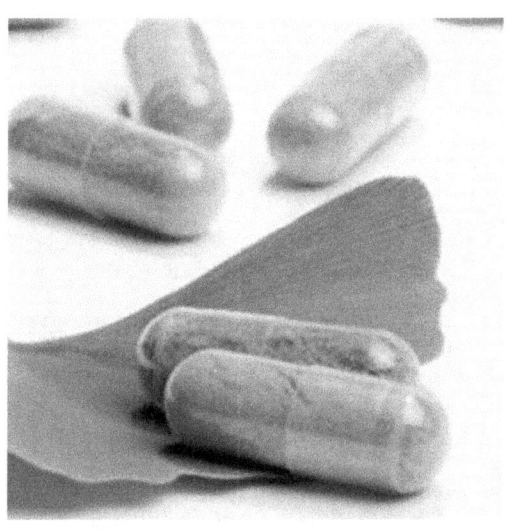

According to the British Medical Journal, a new study confirms that medicinal herbs and natural menopause remedies can be effective and safe treatments for women who want to avoid Hormone Replacement Therapy (HRT), for in some cases it increases risks of breast cancer, heart disease and stroke, among other troubles.

The study revealed that between 50% and 75% of British females in their menopause years have already used natural menopause remedies at least to treat hot flashes and that **soy**, **red clover**, and **black cohosh** effectively reduce perimenopause, menopause and post-menopause symptoms.

These three natural ingredients, by the way, are contained in top over-the-counter menopause relief products including Femestron, which work in a similar way to HRT but with no unwanted side-effects!

WHAT IS MEDICINAL HERBAL THERAPY?

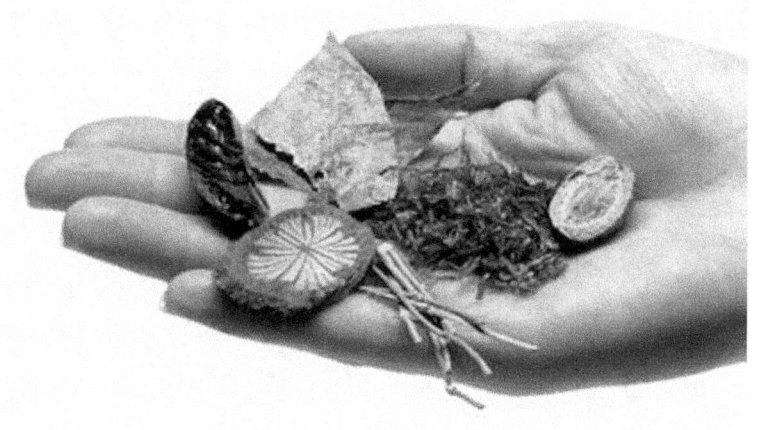

Why are an increasing number of women turning to medicinal herbal therapy to ease their perimenopause, menopause and post-menopause symptoms?

Mainly because for centuries certain herbs have proven to ease menopause symptoms, as stated by the U.S. pharmacist and herbalist Steven G. Ottariano in his best-selling book *Medicinal Herbal Therapy: A Pharmacist's Viewpoint.*

To ease menopause symptoms, Ottariano recommends taking the following medicinal herbs:

Black Cohosh (20 mg to 60 mg, 3 times daily)

Dong Quai (500 mg to 1000 mg, 2 or 3 times daily)

Evening Primrose Oil (500 mg 3 or 4 times daily)

Ginseng (100 mg to 500 mg, 3 times daily)

Vitex Agnus Castus (175 mg daily)

WHAT ARE PLANT ESTROGENS?

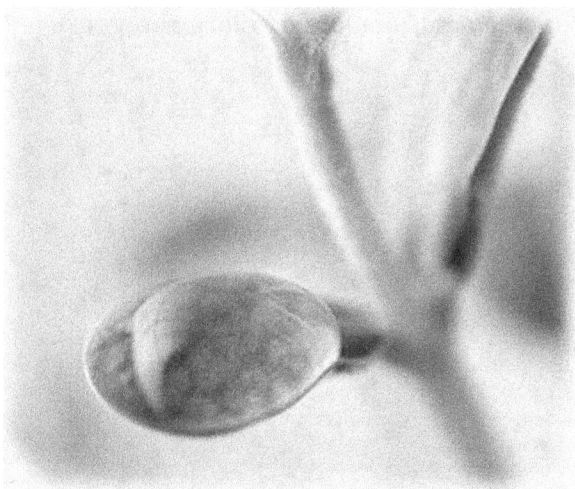

Plant estrogens, popularly known as "dietary estrogens", are contained in phytoestrogenic plants (derived from *phyto* = plant and *estrogen* = fertility hormone produced in female mammals). These nonsteroidal plant compounds are able to produce mild estrogenic effects when taken orally by women.

The most studied belong to the group of substances known as isoflavones, commonly found in phytoestrogenic plants like red clover, soy and lingnans, among others.

Due to their molecular similarities with human estrogen, phytoestrogens have proven to alleviate menopause symptoms. When taken regularly, they reportedly reduce hot flashes and night sweats, among other symptoms.

And the good news is that you can take them orally, either by eating phytoestrogenic-plant foods directly or by taking menopause supplements containing plant estrogens!

CAN WILD YAM HELP REGAIN HORMONAL BALANCE?

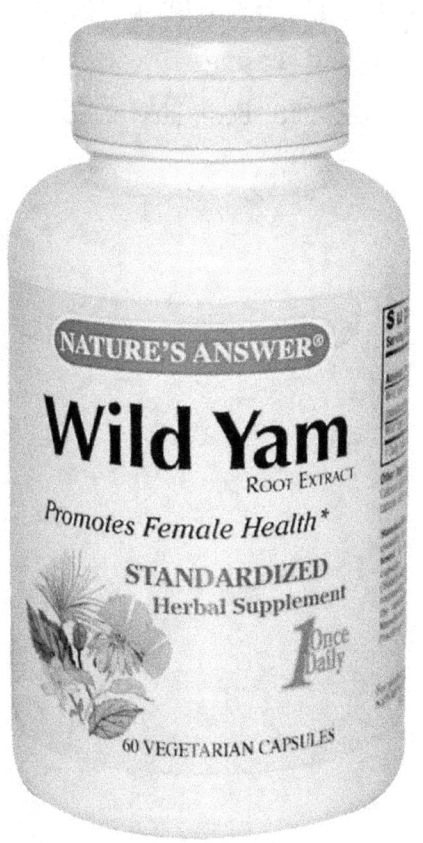

One of the most effective natural ingredients contained in the leading menopause supplements is wild yam *(Dioscorea villosa)*. For centuries, herbalists have used the root of this plant to treat colic, menstrual cramps, and digestive problems, among other disorders, including peri-menopause and menopause symptoms.

Scientific research has shown that wild yam contains diosgenin, a natural substance that can be chemically converted to the hormone progesterone. Taken orally, wild yam is known to increase progesterone levels, helping to reestablish hormonal balance in females and easing a wide range of menopause symptoms with no unwanted secondary effects!

HOW CAN BLACK COHOSH HELP?

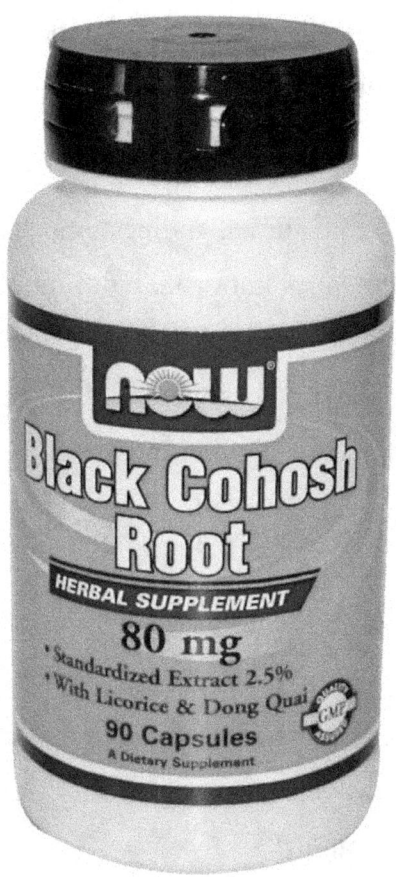

Known by early Americans as "fairy candle", "black snakeroot", and "black bugbane", black cohosh (*actaea racemosa*) is a flowering plant that grows wildly in North American woodlands from Ontario to Georgia, and west to Missouri and Arkansas.

For centuries its root has been one of the most effective natural menopause remedies, traditionally used for treating hot flashes and night sweats along with irritability and restlessness, among other symptoms. Presently, it is one of the main ingredients of the best menopause supplements available on the market, including common over-the-counter remedies.

The Native Americans used it to treat menstrual cramps and hot flashes, as well as sore throat, indigestion, and arthritis, among other affections. We also know that during the Colony it was thought to be the witches brew´s main ingredient and was therefore banned. In fact, in some places women were accused of witchery just for having black cohosh in their possession!

Fortunately times have changed…

Today, black cohosh is one of the main ingredients of the best menopause supplements and over-the-counter remedies (non-prescription and sold online). So, if you´re experiencing hot flashes take black cohosh, proven to ease perimenopause, menopause and post-menopause symptoms!

HOW TO AVOID BRITTLE NAILS?

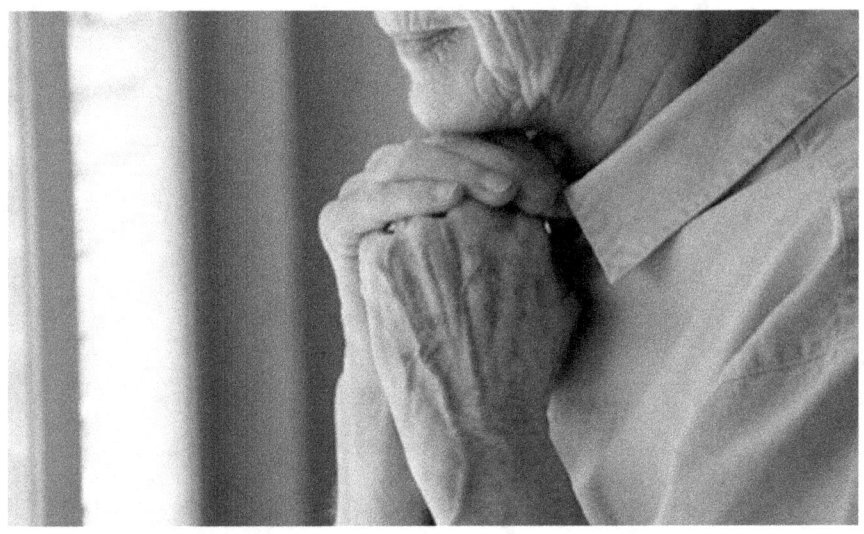

If you are over 40 and your nails are breaking, cracking, splitting or peeling, then you are probably experiencing one of the most-common symptoms of peri-menopause and menopause. Popularly known as "brittle nails", this symptom is caused by a decline in the production of keratin, the hard, structural material of which nails are made of, produced in the outer layer of our skin. This decrease weakens our nails, making it easier for them to break, split, tear or peel.

To avoid brittle nails be sure to take dietary supplements or natural menopause remedies rich in calcium, iron, Vitamin C, folic acid and proteins, which not only increase keratin levels but also tend to balance hormone production.

ARE YOU GROWING HAIRS ON YOUR FACE?

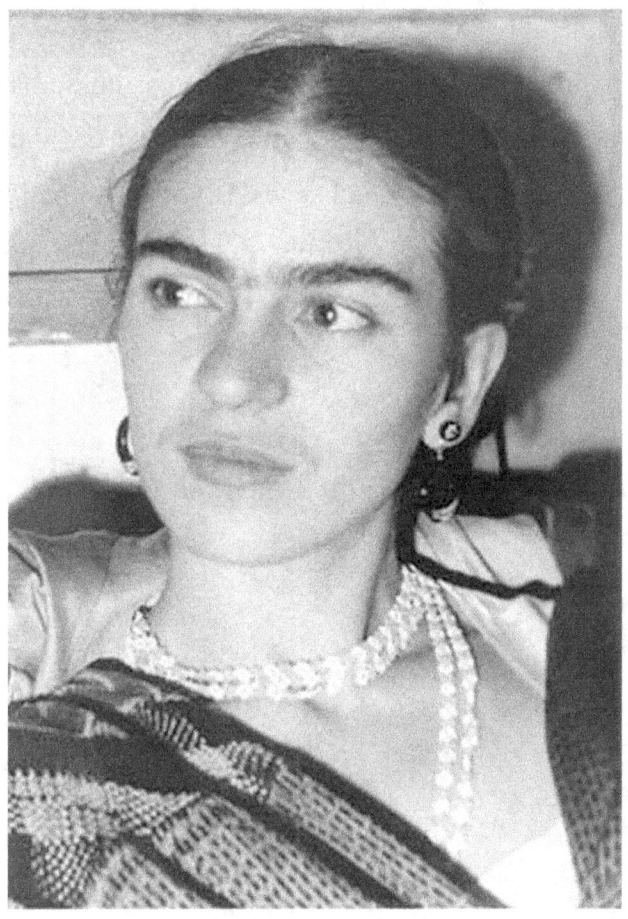

If you are going through menopause and have noticed growing hairs on your upper lip, cheeks, chin, neck, midchest, inner thighs or low back, then you are probably experiencing one of the most unwanted peri-menopause and menopause symptoms. This peculiar symptom is characterized by a "male-pattern hair growth"

and can be compared to a mild form of "hirsutism", a condition mostly found in Mediterranean, Middle Eastern and South Asian women.

To fight this unwanted menopause symptom, a growing number of females are presently relying on therapies based on natural menopause remedies, together with a balanced diet, regular exercise, and healthy lifestyle changes. If you are experiencing this symptom and want help, see your doctor and get professional advice!

HOW TO FIGHT MENOPAUSAL INSOMNIA?

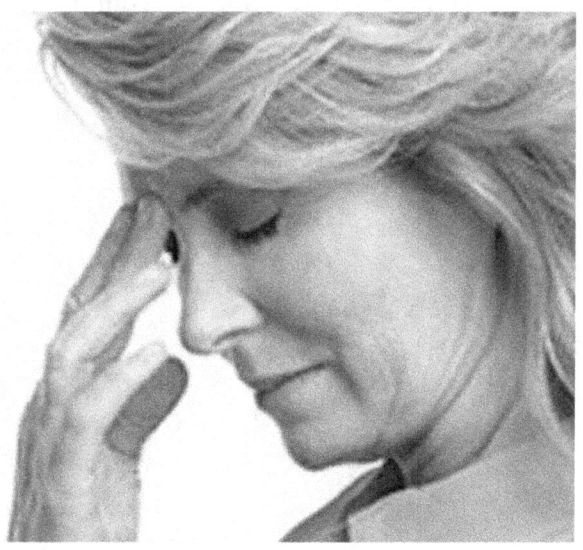

Apart from sleeping pills, there are several alternative treatments worth trying to ease menopausal insomnia. The most recommended are natural products and supplements that include calcium, vitamin D, bisphosphonates. Also recommended are soy products (tofu, soybeans, and soymilk), which contain a plant-hormone similar to estrogen (phytoestrogen); ginseng biloba, as well as red clover and black cohosh extracts, among others.

If you are experiencing difficulties in falling or staying asleep due to hot flashes and night sweat, keep your room cool and well ventilated at nights and try to wear loose clothing to bed –a natural fiber like cotton is recommended. Also recommended is going to bed at the same time each night, according to a regular bedtime schedule. And, before going to bed, avoid excessive caffeine and spicy foods that tend to cause sweating. In any case, if you want to ease these symptoms and improve your sleep, ask your doctor about the benefits of natural supplements and how they can help you regain a normal life.

IS OSTEOPOROSIS CAUSED BY MENOPAUSE?

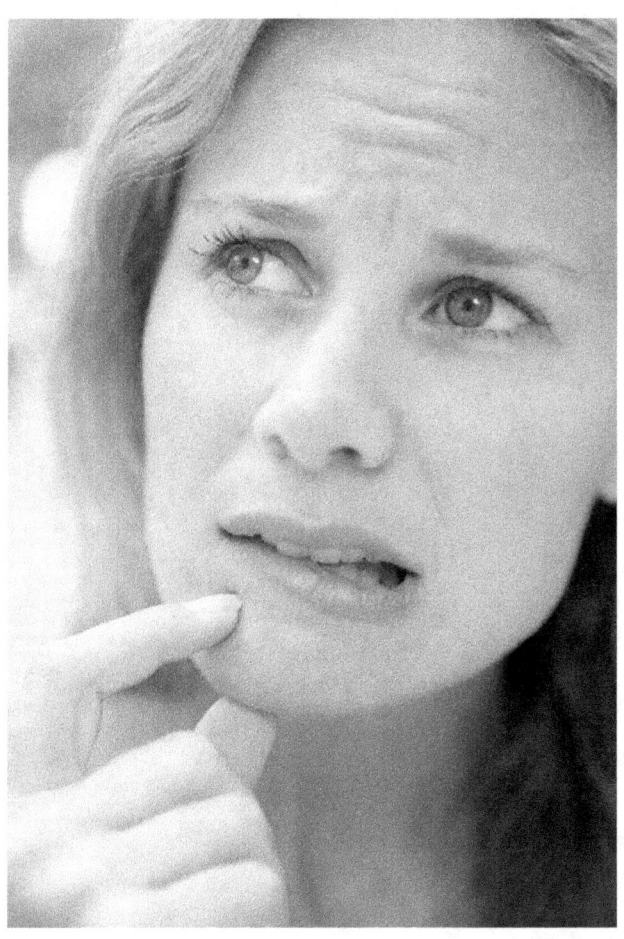

Yes, it is. It is one of the most-feared symptoms of menopause and post-menopause, which means "porous bone". This ailment is also known as "the silent disease" because it usually progresses without any symptoms or pain. It is characterized by gradual loss of bone tissue that weakens them and increases the risk of sudden fractures.

Fortunately, you can prevent osteoporosis and slow down the rate of bone loss by taking menopause supplements containing calcium and vitamin D, as well as by ingesting foods rich in calcium in your daily diet, such as low-fat milk and dairy products, canned fish with bones like sardines and salmon; green leafy vegetables like broccoli and collards, as well as calcium-fortified orange juice and flour, among others. See your doctor for proper treatment!

CAN PROPER **EXERCISE PREVENT**

OSTEOPOROSIS?

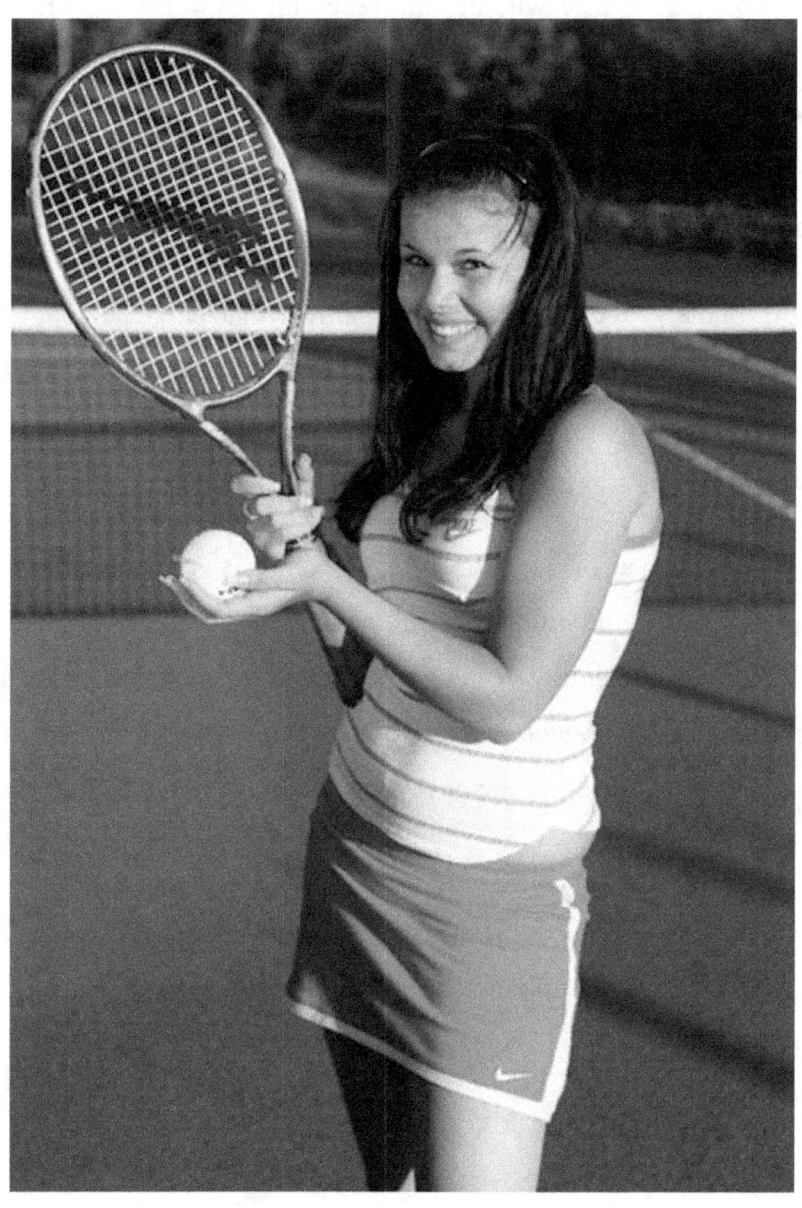

According to the American College of Sports Medicine's *Health and Fitness Journal*, over 25 million people in the U.S. are affected by osteoporosis and most of them (80%) are females in their post-menopause who are not receiving hormone replacement therapy (HRT), don´t take calcium supplements nor exercise regularly. As a result, these women have a 40% fracture risk over their lifetime, with over 1.5 million fractures per year attributed to osteoporosis.

Fortunately, recent studies have shown that exercise programs for women in their post-menopause have increased their bone mineral density (BMD), significantly reducing the risks of osteoporosis.

Although aerobic exercise and weight-bearing activity are important in maintaining overall health, and may contribute to maintenance of healthy bone, resistance exercise seems to have a more significant impact on bone density, together with a balanced diet, a healthy lifestyle plus a regular intake of natural menopause remedies.

In sum, if you are in your post-menopause, exercise regularly, take menopause supplements and see your doctor for proper treatment!

CAN ACUPUNCTURE EASE MENOPAUSE SYMPTOMS?

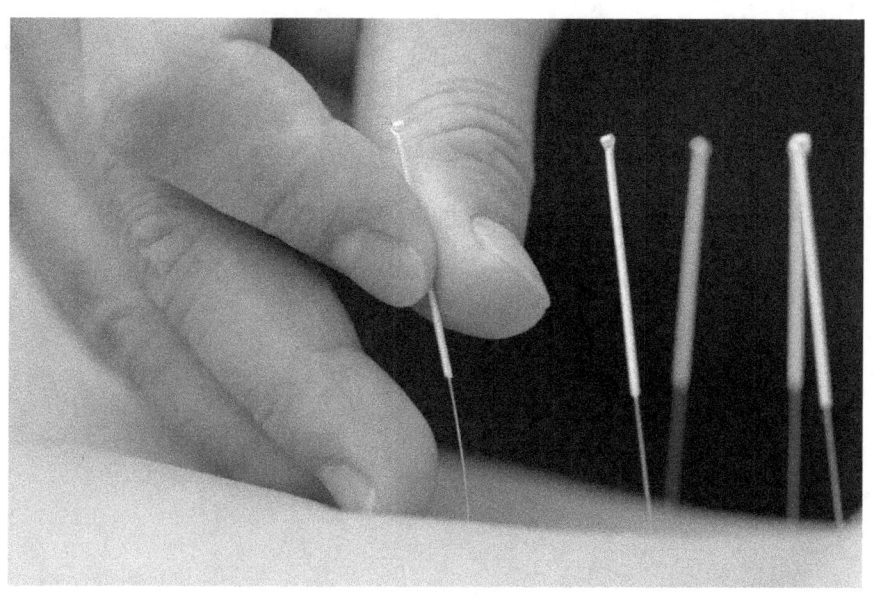

A recent study claims that the ancient Chinese therapy known as "acupuncture" can allegedly help ease some perimenopause, menopause and post-menopause symptoms, including hot flashes and night sweats.

According to the study, published in the *Acupuncture in Medicine* journal, Turkish researchers treated 53 menopausal women with acupuncture and found that the so-called "needle therapy" actually diminishes the frequency and intensity of hot flashes and night sweats, among other symptoms.

Another study from Norway evidenced a reduction in frequency and intensity of hot flashes after using acupuncture for 12 weeks.

Nevertheless, according to the International Menopause Society president David Sturdee, *"the evidence is not strong from previous studies and this is a small trial. We need to have much bigger numbers to prove this really can help women going through the menopause."*

ARE YOU EXPERIENCING A LOSS OF SEX DRIVE?

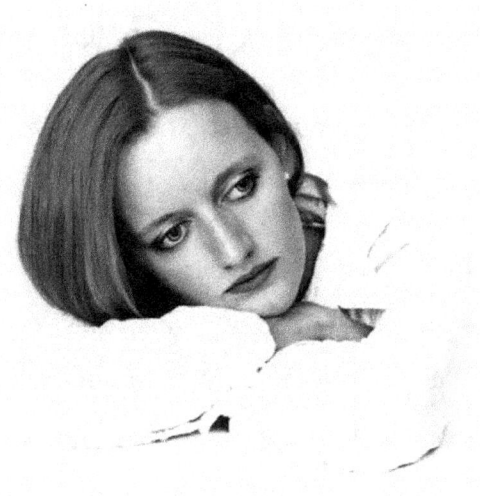

Contrary to what most people believe, sex does not end with menopause.

Although most menopausal women claim to experience a loss of sex drive, in most cases this is not directly caused by the hormonal changes experienced during perimenopause, menopause and post-menopause. In fact, research has shown that menopausal women can enjoy sex as usual if the following conditions are met:

1: Longer foreplays: Most menopausal women experience vaginal dryness. Specialists recommend more cuddling, caressing, massaging and kissing before sex. Prolonged and loving foreplays are always best to get the vaginal juices flowing.

2:End foreplay with direct stimulation: Foreplay should always end with direct stimulation of the vaginal area (orally or manually). If manual, always use vaginal lubricants.

3 Use lubricants during penetration: To ease penetration and avoid pain use vaginal lubricants (KY jelly or similar).

For most married women, marital sex is vital to keep a relationship alive. This view was the basis of a recent survey conducted by the online women's community iVillage with the participation of 1,001 wives ages 18-49. The survey showed that 75% of the participants admitted that sharing a good sex life with their couple is "very or extremely important". On the other hand, only 16% of them considered marital sex "somewhat important." The survey also found that the main reasons for not wanting sex are stress, exhaustion, children, lack of romance, arguments and loss of physical attraction.

In the case of women in their mid-40s and older, we should include another set of important reasons for not wanting sex: the undesirable effects of perimenopause, menopause, and post-menopause. These three stages in a woman's life, also known as "The Change", are produced from a natural drop in the production of hormones like estrogen and progesterone, which regulate fertility, menstruation, procreation and maternity, therefore affecting a wide number of bodily functions.

Pain during intercourse seems to be the main reason for most of women who lose interest in sex during "The Change". This pain is generally caused by vaginal dryness (derived from thinner vaginal lining), causing difficulties and maltreatment during sexual intercourse.

Researchers have found conflicting results regarding estrogen replacement therapy as a treatment for vaginal dryness. In turn, most doctor recommend the use of lubricants (like K-Y jelly, for example) as well as estrogen creams, which lubricate and restore the lining's thickness and consistency when applied vaginally.

During "The Change", it must be said, sexual performance can also be affected by hot flashes, night sweats, brain fog, mood swings, irritability, depression, and headaches, among others. If you are experiencing some or all of these symptoms, my advice is to wake up and take a stand. Find out all you can about the different therapies available and please consult your physician!

EXPERIENCING THE EMPTY NEST SYNDROME?

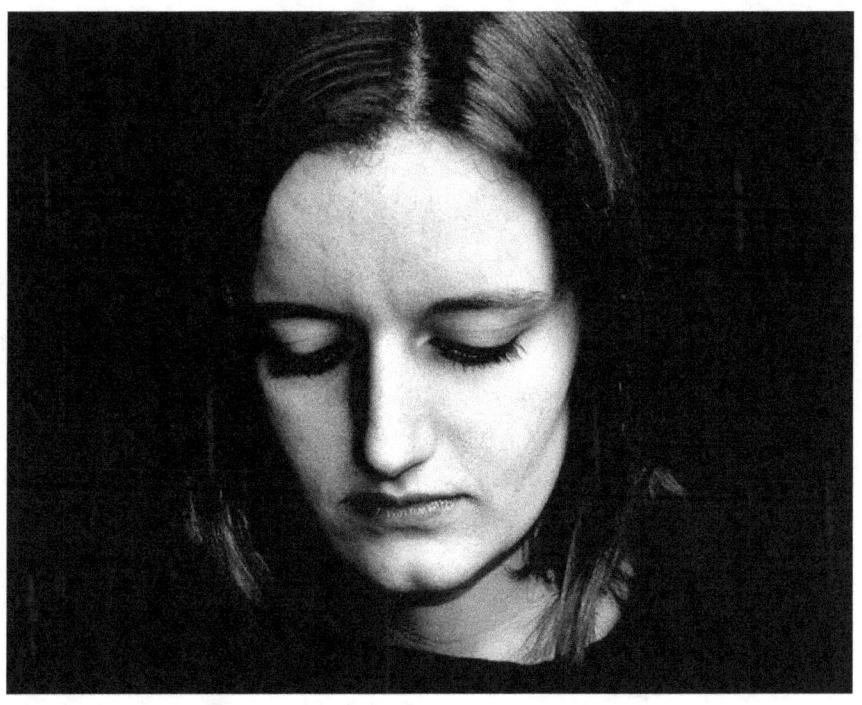

Depression can be one of your worst menopause symptoms, especially if you're experiencing what specialists call the "Empty Nest Syndrome", often described as *"a feeling of loss, sadness and loneliness experienced by parents when their children grow up and leave home."*

According to *Psychology Today*'s Diagnosis Dictionary, the Empty Nest Syndrome often causes depression, sadness, and/or grief. Mothers are more likely to be affected than fathers by the departure of their children. Especially because most mothers, as they reach this stage, also happen to be going through the stages of menopause.

Keeping an active and productive life seems to alleviate the feeling of loss and emptiness caused by separation, as well as taking natural menopause supplements, maintaining a balanced diet, exercising regularly and keeping healthy habits.

If you're experiencing the Empty Nest Syndrome and are in your perimenopause, menopause or post-menopause, consider seeing your doctor for professional help!

TURNING MENOPAUSE INTO A NEW BEGINNING?

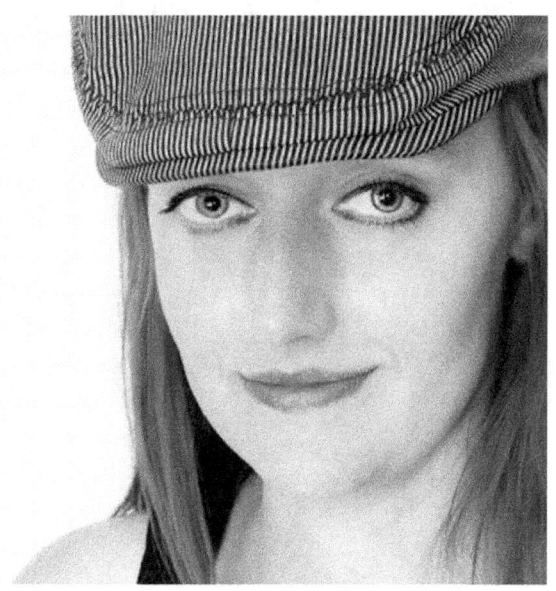

My best friend Diana couldn't stand being menopausal! I talked to her for months, told her it was not the end and that she was not alone. In fact, millions of women are presently coping with menopause and, fortunately, there are new treatments now, as well as innovative **menopause relief products** proven to ease its symptoms.

Everything changed the day Diana went to see her doctor and started her treatment, which not only included natural menopause remedies, but also regular exercise, a balanced diet, and adopting healthier lifestyle habits.

Now, six months later, Diana actually believes menopause is "*a new beginning*" and, quoting Oprah Winfrey, she claims it's "*your moment to reinvent yourself after years of focusing on the needs of everyone else. It's your opportunity to get clear about what matters to you and then to pursue that with all of your energy, time and talent...*"

WHAT IS POSTMENOPAUSAL ZEST?

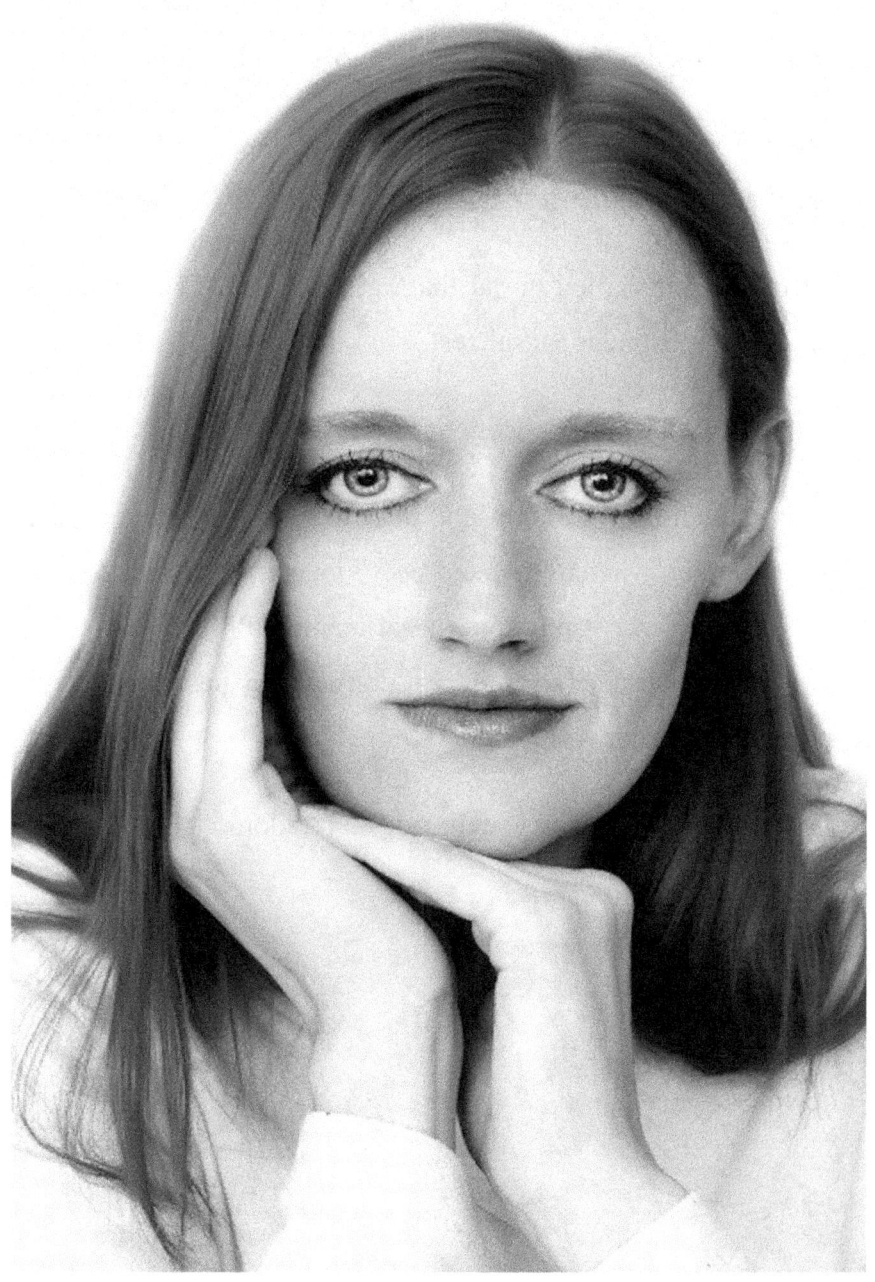

On February 19, 1970, "The David Frost Show" presented an interview with the sixty-nine-year-old anthropologist Margaret Mead (1901-78), author of **Sex and Temperament in Three Primitive Societies** (1935) and **Male and Female** (1949).

When Frost asked Margaret Mead how she managed to keep up a pace that would exhaust females half her age, she answered:

"It might have killed me at that age –she said-. I attribute my energy to my postmenopausal zest."

On that day the term "postmenopausal zest" was first coined.

Ever since it has been in use to describe the enthusiastic feeling experienced by women in their post-menopause, when they no longer need to worry about menstrual cramps, PMS, birth control, and other female inconveniences normally experienced before reaching their menopause.

"This", Margaret Mead concluded, "is freedom."

THANKS FOR READING THIS BOOK!

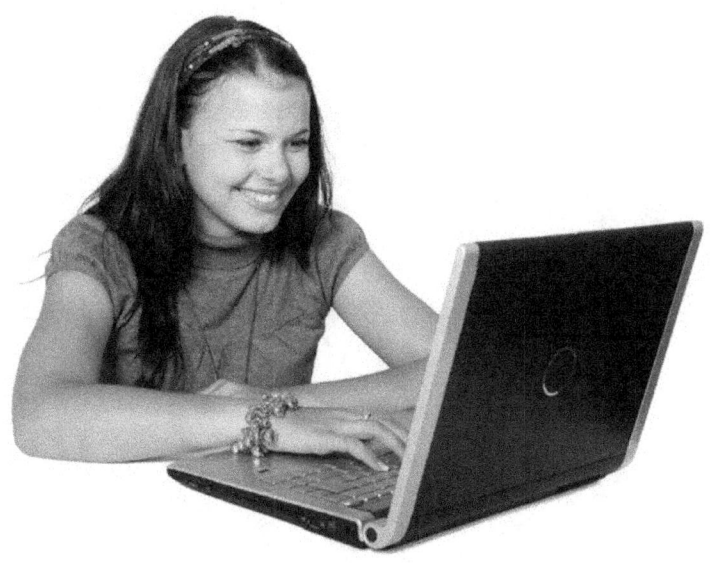

If you found this book helpful, please consider taking a few moments to leave your REVIEW on Amazon!

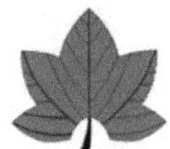

Vermont Indie Books

2015

www.ingramcontent.com/pod-product-compliance
Lightning Source LLC
Chambersburg PA
CBHW072015290526
45787CB00013B/916